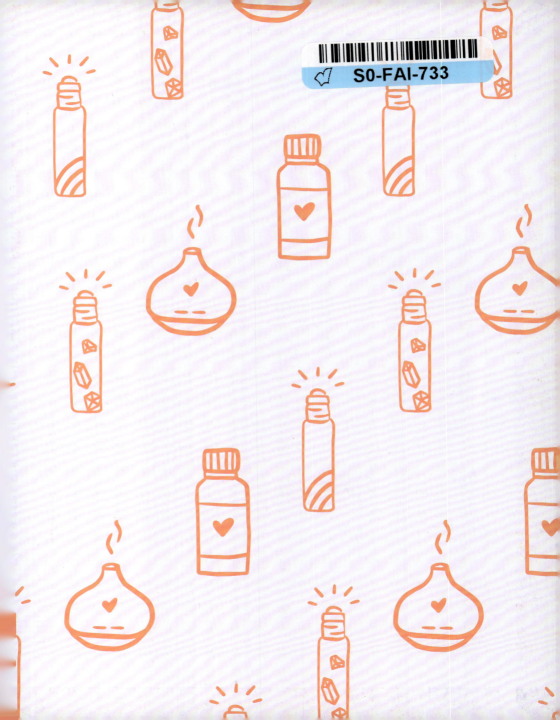

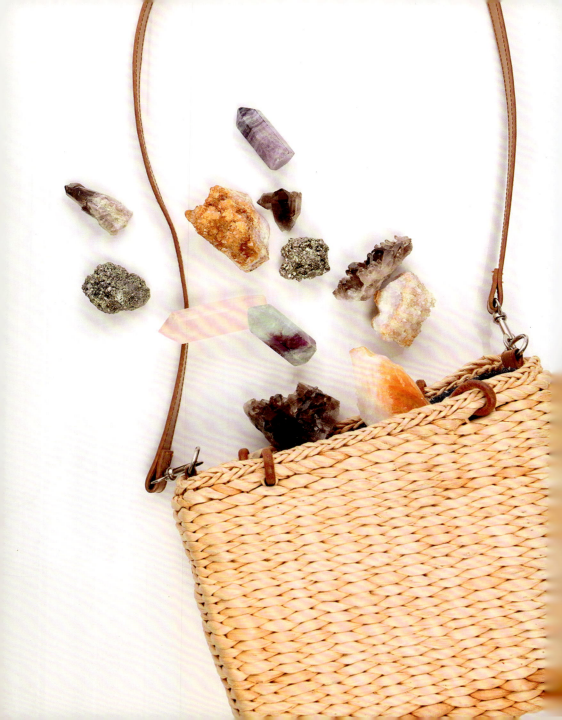

Table of contents

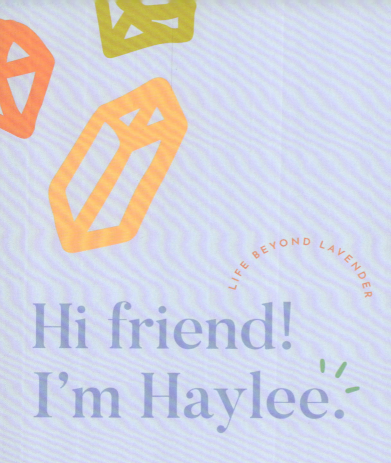

Hi friend! I'm Haylee.

I have three kids and my husband and I run Whimsy + Wellness which I started myself—like what? I still don't believe it most days. My personal mantra is that wellness should be happy. I mean, isn't joy the point of being well?

If you're tired of all those little essential oil bottles piling up in your drawers and bathroom shelves, this book will help you break out of your rut and embrace the fun in wellness again.

These pages are filled with whimsy and joy; just between you and me, this may be the most fun you've ever had with wellness!

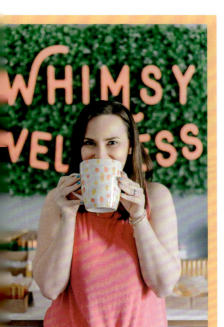

THAT OIL STASH THO..

How did your oily story begin? Mine got its start in 2014. I was trying to save a few dollars by making my own Christmas gifts for friends and family, and I wanted to scent them naturally. A friend invited me over for dinner, showed me her oil stash, and the rest was history.

It didn't take long for me to discover the power of a good essential oil recipe. These simple little blends have helped me sleep, smile on rainy days—and make the BEST perfumes.

THE RAINBOWS AFTER THE RAIN

Essential oil recipes also helped console and heal me after 2 heartbreaking miscarriages. In fact, it was creating roller bottles for my recipes that distracted me from the pain, which in turn led to Whimsy + Wellness.

I wasn't enchanted by any of the rollers I was finding, so I made my own and began sharing them with others. They've been flying off our shelves ever since. We are truly the lucky ones.

My husband Russ and I have two beautiful rainbow babies now (and my 9 year old stepson!), and Whimsy + Wellness has grown into an amazing community. We talk about loss, love, and grief—and always find the joy in the everyday.

If there's one thing I know, it's the power of a good roller bottle or diffuser recipe. Trust me, there's an essential oil adventure waiting for you beyond lavender ;).

POWER TO THE PEOPLE

How to use your oils safely

I don't enjoy this part but I have to get it out: the tragic truth is that the products we rely on to help our families (baby shampoo, conditioner, soap, etc.) aren't well regulated, and there's a lot we don't know about what's lurking inside.

What we do know is that they contain a lot of nasty stuff—everything from toxic, cancer-causing chemicals to ingredients that disrupt our endocrine systems (your thyroid and hormones) and impact our children's growth and development*.

BUT DON'T PANIC, KAREN! This page is about to get a lot happier! That's the power of essential oils—they put the power back into our hands so we can take charge of our health and wellness, know what's in our cosmetics and household supplies, and enjoy the good life with no weird or disturbing side effects in sight.

KNOWLEDGE IS POWER

A quality essential oil company will label your bottle with clear use instructions. Pay attention to them, and consult experienced oil users like the person who signed you up when you began your oil journey!

Here are some tips for using your oils safely

- If you have sensitive skin, test a tiny patch of your skin before you treat a larger area
- Avoid your eyes
- Be very careful applying oils to young children—some oils should never be used for little ones
- For the littlest oilers, start by wearing oils on yourself, then diffusing oils in the room, and then—once kids are over the age of 2—you can use them topically, but only when they're very diluted
- When in doubt, dilute—some people will always need to dilute more than others

PETS + OILS

Most pets' noses are way more powerful than yours, so make sure Fido can leave the room when you start diffusing. He'll leave if it gets to be too much for him. And talk to your vet before using essential oil topically for him.

Interested in doing your own research? EWG.org is a great place to start!

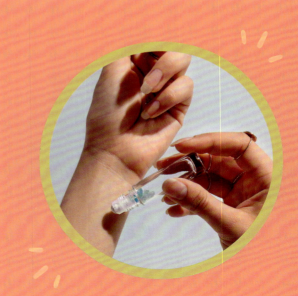

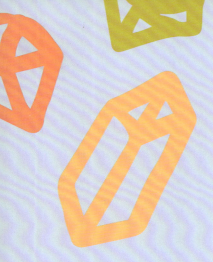

How to dilute your oils

That little bottle of earthy, oily goodness in your hand? Don't make the mistake of thinking that just because it's natural, you can use it all willy nilly. These natural resources are potent!

Don't be scared, though. Your intuition is powerful—you know what's best for yourself and your family. Plus, you have dilution on your side! And here are my best tips for tapping into its power.

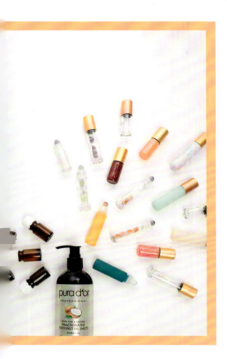

WHY DILUTE

Dilution helps you tap into your amazing little oil friends without harming anybody's sensitive skin. Plus, some oils are pretty pricey (*side eye to rose*) diluting them with a carrier oil means you'll save money by not having to buy oils as often.

But my favorite reason to dilute oils? It means I'll grab my oils more frequently. Diluting means I'm whipping up roller bottles, dropper bottles, and spray bottles with my favorite blends so they are easily accessible.

I'm not above using oils directly on skin (I always make sure to test them first), but I'm also not about to go fumbling in random drawers for an oil that may or may not work. Instead, I'm the superhero with the oil power at my fingertips thanks to my on-hand recipes and my roller bottles!

FRACTIONED COCONUT OIL FTW

My absolute favorite carrier oil to dilute with is fractionated coconut oil. The kind I get has a pump, so adding it to roller bottles is easy. In fact, simply diluting the oil in my hand is also easy in a pinch!. You can also use jojoba oil, olive oil, sweet almond oil, and vitamin E oil (sweet almond oil and vitamin E oil are great for facial application!).

Here's a pro tip: the sniff test doesn't always work, friends. Label your bottles!

The charts below are conservative estimates, and great places to start. Feel like you need something more powerful? You do you, boo!

How do I dilute for...	Good for...
1% Dilution	Children 2 and up, the elderly, sensitive skin, facial use, and/or long-term daily use
2% Dilution	Healthy adults with regular use
3% Dilution	Treatment for pain or discomfort over short periods of time

What about my diffuser?

To keep a diffuser blend on hand, fill a dropper bottle with your favorite oils to diffuse together, shake well before use, then add a few drops of your special blend directly to your diffuser. You can also just add drops directly from your oil bottles.

Your diffuser should have instructions for your oil to water ratio, but a typical ratio is 3-5 drops per 100ml of water. Don't know what size your diffuser is? Not to worry! I like to do 5 drops to start. If I want a stronger scent, I'll turn the diffuser off and add a few more drops. Don't be afraid to experiment to find what works for you.

Popular Diffuser Sizes
100ml = 3-5 drops
300ml = 9-15 drops
500ml = 15-25 drops

DILUTION GUIDE FOR ROLLER OR DROPPER BOTTLES

Bottle size	Intended use	Number of drops
5 ml	2-5 years	1-3 drops
	5-12 years	3-5 drops
	13+ years	7-10 drops
	Extra strength	10+ drops
10 ml	2-5 years	2-5 drops
	5-12 years	5-10 drops
	13+ years	15-20 drops
	Extra strength	20+ drops

How to pair crystals with your blends

Do crystals give off a hippie vibe? Yes. Are they also so mouthwateringly beautiful? Yes. Am I a hippie? Probably.

Crystals are ancient little nuggets of love and beauty from the earth, and they pair beautifully with essential oil blends. *chef's kiss* Here's a little more on how to use them with your oils!

IT'S SCIENCE

If you love essential oils, you already know there's a whole world of wellness outside of modern medical journals. We are just relearning to tap into it, like our ancestors did thousands of years ago.

Science tells us crystals have a crystalline structure that gives off measurable energy. Unlike your energy and my energy which changes and gets wacky all the time, crystals' energies are constant (ever heard of crystal components used in watches to tell time?).

Crystals bring our energies back into balance and alignment—that's what people mean when they talk about the healing power of crystals.

YOUR BODY KNOWS

Pairing crystals and oils isn't rocket science (thank heavens). The more you get in touch with your own intuition, the more you'll find yourself instinctively drawn to the crystals and oils you need. Your body is smart—listen to her and let her be your guide.

If that's a little too woo-woo, start with a symptom you want to heal or an intention you want to set. Struggling with anxiety? Insomnia? Want to welcome an abundance mindset or peaceful vibes into your home? Choose a crystal that helps, and then a corresponding blend from our handy dandy chart on the next page.

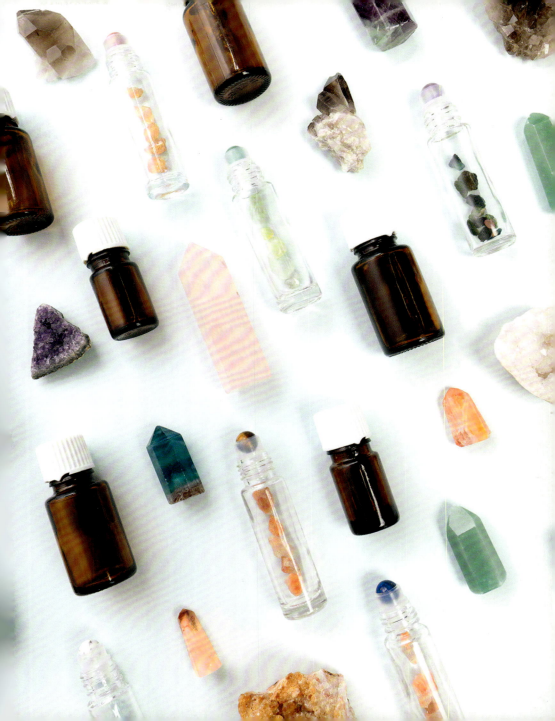

And if you want to pair a crystal with an oil recipe that's not a "match?" I'm not judging—you can't do this wrong, friend. If it makes you smile, you're winning!

Crystal	Good for...	Recipe
Amazonite	Courage and truth, dispels negative energy, worry, and fear	Some Dadgum Peace & Quiet (p. 53), Tastes Like Cotton Candy (p. 65)
Amethyst	A good overall stone, can be used for protection, balance, and help with confidence	I Believe (p. 36), I Dream of Naps (p. 44), Mommy Needs You to Go Night Night (p. 52), Extra Flowers, Please (p. 56), Calm Down (p. 58), The Magic Wand (p. 53), TGI Summer (p. 58), Be Well, My Friend (p. 59)
Aquamarine	Courage, calms the mind, useful for closure, promotes self-expression	Zen, Baby (p. 36)
Aventurine	Release self-destructive patterns, a relationship stone, embrace daily joy	Breathing is Nice (p. 44), Bye, Pollen (p. 56), I'd Rather Be Outside (p. 49)
Bloodstone	Healing, realigning, balancing	Moms Don't Get Sick Roller Blend (p. 44)
Blue lace agate	Speaking your truth, increasing clarity, bringing mind and heart into alignment	Peace (p. 36), The Great Outdoors is My Spa (p. 41)
Carnelian	Creativity, joy, abundance	Pixie Dust (p. 37), She Fierce (p. 45), Working All Day and Night Energy (p. 48), Give Me Energy (p. 45), Leave the Work at the Office (p. 49), We So Bougie (p. 65)
Chrysocolla	Communication, teaching stone, encourages compassion, peace, and forgiveness	Ahhhhh Cooling Mist (p. 58)
Citrine	Success, abundance, creativity, power	Smile Real Big (p. 36), How You Doin' Cologne Spray (p. 48), I Love This Home (p. 59), Big Presentation Vibes (p. 49), Vacation in a Bottle (p. 58), Coming Up Lemons Counter Top Spray (p. 65)
Clear quartz	An ultimate healer, amplifies whatever energy or intent is programmed to it	Trust the Process (p. 37), Manly Man Beard Oil (p. 48), Man Flu (p. 49), No Sick Here (p. 52), Nama Stay Zen (p. 41), Baths Aren't Just for Girls Bath Salts Blend (p. 49)
Dalmation stone	Brings out the child in us, encourages a sense of humor and playfulness, a grounding and calming energy, a pick-me-up stone	All the Sleep You Need Glow Serum (p. 41)
Garnet	Positive stone, uplifting, inspires love and devotion	I Wish (For No More Laundry) (p. 37), Jingle All the Way (p. 60)
Hematite	Grounding, connecting, increasing self-confidence	I Work Out (p. 44), Best Night's Sleep of Your Life (p. 48), Let's See Those Muscles (p. 48), Spicy Spray (p. 59), Everybody is Stressin' Me Out (p. 45)

Crystal	Good for...	Recipe
Jade	Purification, gentle support and nourishment	Normal Skin Serum (p. 40), Skin Magic (p. 45), My Manly Face Needs Soothing Skin Serum (p. 49)
Lapis Lazuli	Wisdom, good judgement, desire for knowledge, stone of truth	Dry Skin Serum (p. 41)
Pink opal	Stone of renewal, calming, emotional balance	Chase the Rainbow Perfume Spray (p. 37), Problems? What Problems? Bath Salts Blend (p. 41), Get My Sleep on Spray (p. 45)
Rainbow fluorite	Increasing harmony and focus, tapping into your intuitive abilities	I Can Do Math in My Head (p. 44), Please Do Your Homework (p. 52), Too Many Zoom Meetings (p. 64)
Rose quartz	The ultimate love and relationships stone	I Am My Favorite Person Perfume Spray (p. 37), Oily Or Acne-Prone Skin Serum (p. 41), Lights (p. 60), I Sing My Own Love Songs (p. 45), We're Both Learning Here (p. 53)
Rhodonite	Reconciliation, healing emotional wounds and past trauma	Happy Happy Happy (p. 36), Because I'm (Trying to Be) Happy (p. 52), Perky (p. 56)
Ruby	Energy, love stone, increases concentration and motivation	New Year, I'm Perfect Perfume Spray (p. 60)
Selenite	Greater harmony and balance with inner self, cleansing	Bye, Mystery Smell (p. 65), I Just "Cleaned" My House (p. 64)
Smoky quartz	Detoxifying, blocking negative energy, settling fears	OMG It's Fall (p. 59), Treat Every Day Like Christmas (p. 60), Ya'll, It's Cold Out There (p. 60), Bug Off Spray (p. 58), Zen & Cozy (p. 59), THAT Candle (You Know the One) (p. 65)
Sunstone (or tiger's eye)	Leadership, joyful stone, inspires nurturing of self	Sunshine in My Pocket (p. 36), Hear Me Roar (p. 37), Pepto But Better (p. 44), Tummy Probs (p. 52), Make Me Smell Like Pumpkin Spice (p. 59), I'm Not a Baker (But I Play One on TV) (p. 60)
Topaz	Good fortune, goals, luck	Teeth are the WORST (p. 53)
Tourmaline	Promotes understanding of self, attracts inspiration, compassion	No More Monsters Under the Bed Room Spray (p. 53), S'mores (p. 58)
White howlite	Increase wonder and excitement, decrease frustration and anger	Who Says Men Can't Have Spa Days (p. 48), We've Lost That Calm Feeling (p. 52)

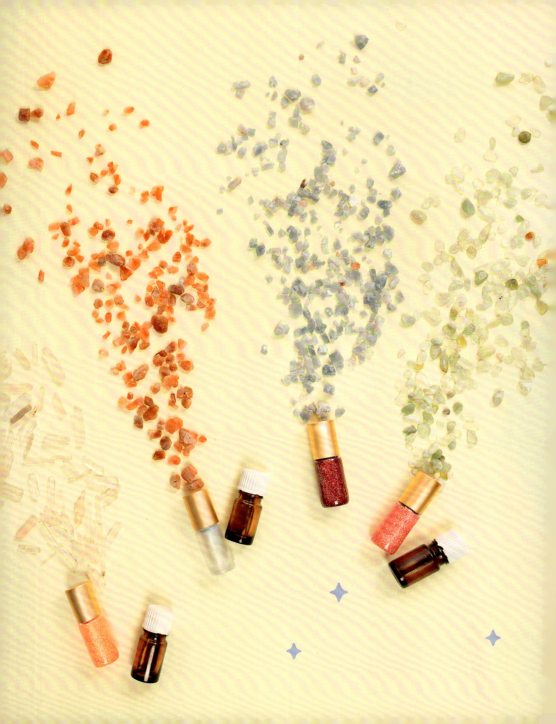

Crystals come in different sizes and shapes

- Large enough to sit on a shelf or wherever you'll see them often
- Small and smooth enough to slip into your pocket for a day (or even under your pillow at night)
- Integrated into jewelry
- Held in your hand, usually while you're meditating or setting an intention for the day

Here are some things you can do with the oils

- Diffuse them in a diffuser
- Roll them onto pulse points using a roller bottle
- Use a spray bottle and make room sprays, linen sprays, or cleaning solutions
- Drop them in a bath
- Add drops to a strip of leather or wool to serve as tiny, wearable diffusers

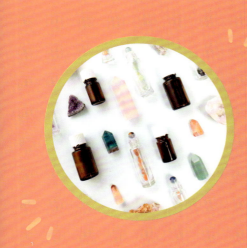

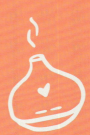

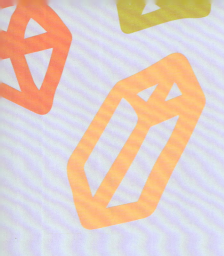

So much oil love

I love using crystals and I love using essential oils—and I really love using them together. Here are a few of my favorite ways to do that:

DIFFUSER KITS

Keep a diffuser + a dropper bottle with your favorite diffuser recipe + your favorite crystal on a shelf or tabletop in several rooms in your house.

In the morning, add cheerful, focus, or cozy diffuser recipes to the diffusers in the main rooms of your house (kitchen, living room, etc.). In the evening, add sleepy time recipes to the diffusers in the bedrooms.

GEMSTONE MORNINGS

Roll a gemstone roller bottle filled with your favorite daily perfume on the inside of your wrists and the back of your neck when you wake up in the morning. Throw open the blinds, welcome the sun, breathe deeply, and set your intention for the day.

CRYSTAL MEDITATION

Use an app like Headspace or Dwell to meditate during the day. Diffuse a peaceful, calming oil blend and hold your favorite crystal in your hand while you practice.

GEMS ON THE GO

Slip crystals into clear glass rollers so that they're always ready for your favorite essential oils recipes. When you feel the need for a new blend, consult our handy dandy chart above. Roll, smile, feel well.

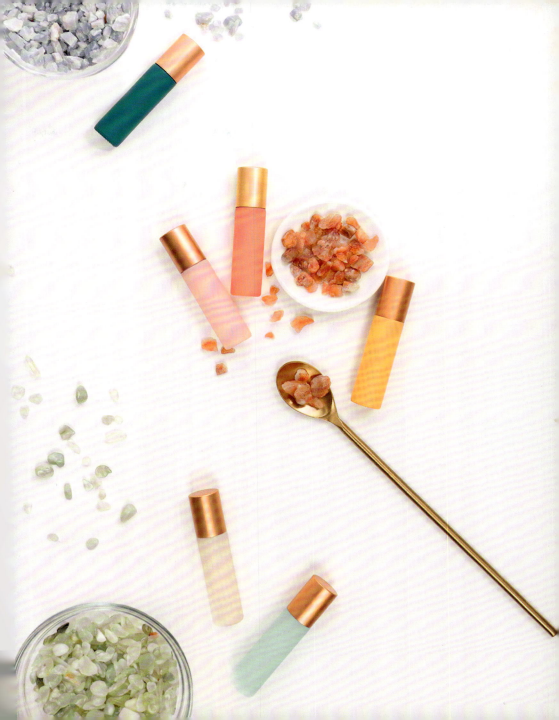

Your oils never smelled so good

There are some things essential oils can't do.

They can, for example, make your kitchen smell like rosemary and a lemon orchard, but eventually you're going to have to put all those coffee mugs into the dishwasher, boo.

Essential oils *can* help you sleep like a baby at night, but they're not bringing you breakfast in bed followed by a Swedish massage and a Target shopping spree. I'm sad about this too.

But you know what essential oils can do?

They can make you smell amazing. Like, "I woke up like this" amazing. Effortless, "who, me?" amazing. Hasn't showered in days, hair is 99% dry shampoo, wearing yesterday's clothes, but I still smell *divine* kind of amazing.

A custom perfume blend by way of essential oils is exactly the beauty pick-me-up you've been looking for, and I don't care if you're more the Chanel No. 5 type or the unwashed hippie type. There's a custom essential oil perfume *just* for you.

The best news? It's not difficult.

Here's what you need to know:

LET'S MAKE SOME (PERFUME) MUSIC!

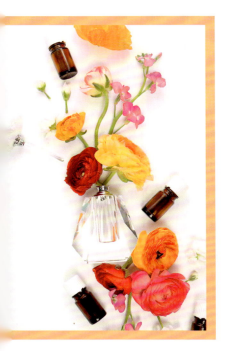

Scents are exciting and complex! When you're using essential oils to create scents, you're not only getting the benefits of non-toxic beauty (fragrance is some of the most toxic beauty stuff you can buy) AND the benefits of aromatherapy.

In other words, even if nothing else goes your way all day, your perfume roller will still have your back.

When you're creating perfumes, pay attention to how the aromas sit with you. The top note is the smell you experience first. Citrus is almost always a top note because it gets straight to business. It's bright and clear.

Middle notes are the heart of the perfume—the solid, respectable middle. They carry the perfume.

Base notes are the foundation of the whole thing. They give it verve and strength and some lingering action, since they're the last thing you smell.

When you create a perfume, you'll choose a top note, one or two middle notes, and one or two base notes. Use my chart below; it's really that simple.

Two tips for you

- Ditch the "rules" whenever you feel like it. This is your perfume—you get to decide what smells good
- Take the lids off the oils you're thinking about combining, and sort of run all the bottles by your nose at the same time. Do you like them together? You'll probably like them as a perfume.

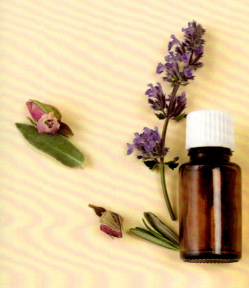

Top notes

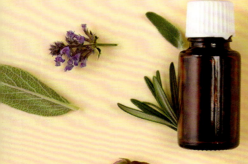

Middle notes

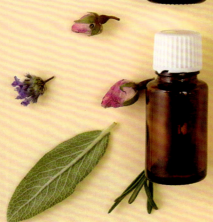

Base notes

NEED AN EXAMPLE? I GOTCHA!

The charts below will take your perfume skills to Paris-perfumery levels. Once you've added the suggested number of oil drops, add your carrier oil (fractionated coconut oil is odorless and ideal for this) and the roller top and you're done!

See? So easy. But if you need an example, here's mine:

Perfumes are super fun to make for friends as gifts. Let's say you're making a blend for a friend who abhors ultra-feminine scents. You might start by choosing earthy and woodsy scents like patchouli as a base note and cypress or pine as the middle notes. These scent families pair well together and are generally crowd-pleasers.

When it comes to the top note, you can stay in the same scent families, or you might look for something in the citrus family, because it pairs so well with almost everything and will help lighten and brighten those darker, moodier scents. I love bergamot. It's a sophisticated citrus scent that makes a great top note!

Once I've picked my scents and done the sniff test to make sure I like the combo, I'll start adding them to my roller bottle. To make my friend's perfume, I'll use about 4 drops of patchouli as my base note, 12 drops of cypress or pine as my middle note, and 4 drops bergamot as my top note. Voila!

PS- You can totally put perfumes in spray bottles too! I recommend using vodka instead of carrier oil after adding in your essential oils. I know it sounds weird, but I promise you don't smell the vodka at all, and it evaporates quickly leaving just the essential oils' scent on you.

PPS- The chart on the next page is for a stronger scented perfume (the way I like it, but to each their own!) so feel free to play around with the numbers to find the strength that works for you! Annnnd you can always do a little math to make these ratios match any size bottle you're working with.

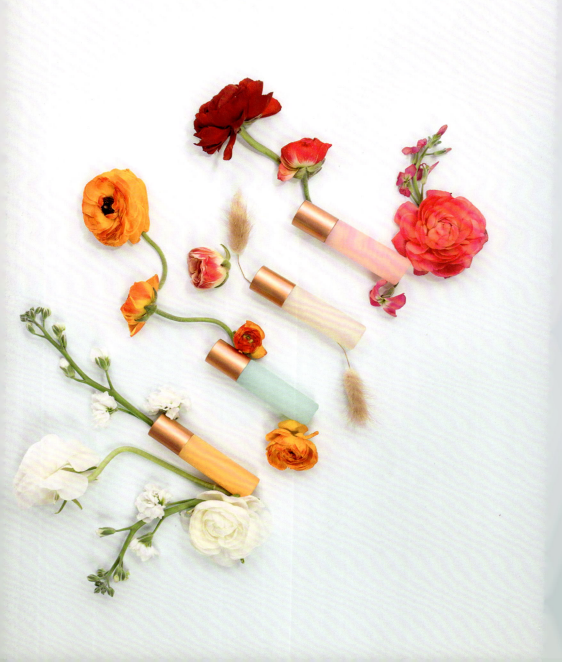

Notes	% of blend	5 ml	10 ml
Top notes	20-40%	4-8 drops	8-16 drops
Middle notes	40-80%	8-16 drops	16-32 drops
Base notes	10-25%	2-5 drops	4-10 drops

FLORAL FAMILY

Floral Family (blends well with spicy, citrus, and woodsy scent families)

Top notes	Middle notes
Lavender	Chamomile
	Geranium
	Ylang ylang

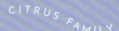

CITRUS FAMILY

Citrus Family (almost always a top note; blends well with almost any other oil)

Top notes	
Orange	Lime
Lemon	Tangerine
Grapefruit	Bergamot
Jade lemon	Citronella
Lemongrass	

MINTY FAMILY

Minty Family (blends well with citrus, woodsy, herby, and earthy scent families)

Top notes	
Spearmint	Wintergreen
Peppermint	

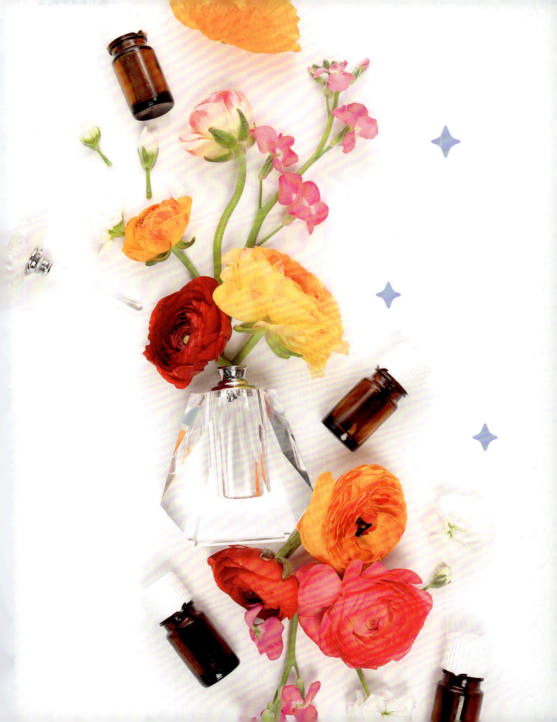

Herby Family (blends well with minty, citrus, woodsy, and earthy scent families)

Top notes	Middle notes
Basil	Thyme
	Rosemary
	Fennel

Earthy Family (blends well with floral, woodsy, and citrus scent families)

Base notes	
Patchouli	Frankincense
Vetiver	Copaiba

SPICY FAMILY

Spicy Family (blends well with floral and citrus scent families)

Top notes	Middle notes	Base notes
Coriander	Clove	Ginger
Cinnamon	Cardamom	
	Black Pepper	
	Nutmeg	

WOODSY FAMILY

Woodsy Family (generally blends well with everything)

Top notes	Middle notes	Base notes
Eucalyptus	Tea tree	Idaho balsam fir
Sage	Cypress	Cedarwood
	Juniper	
	Spruce	
	Myrtle	
	Pine	
	Palo santo	

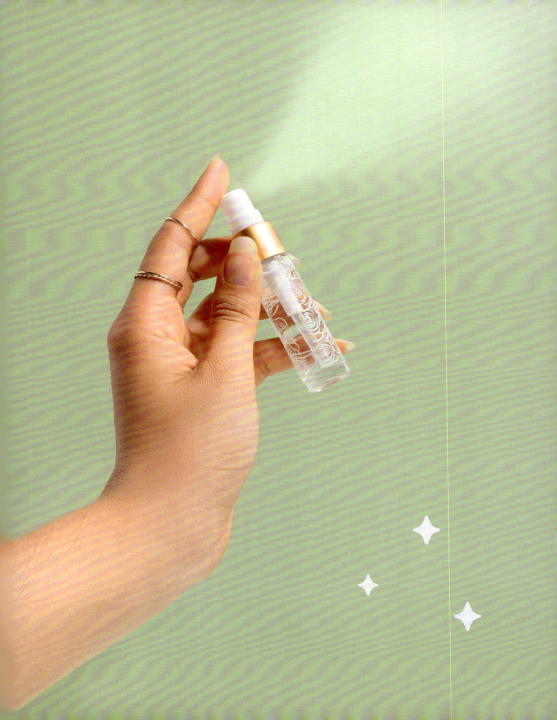

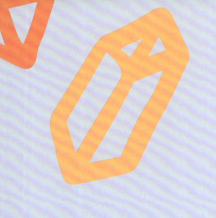

Recipes for dayssss

Are you ready for this? These are the best Whimsy + Wellness recipes. Use them, love them—and when you snap an Instagram pic to show your friends how great they are, don't forget to tag us (@whimsyandwellness) so we can do a happy dance right along with you.

SUBSTITUTIONS

Sometimes we get asked—which fir do I use? Which eucalyptus? And let me tell you, it's whichever one is your favorite! Any of them will work, and I have a feeling if you choose your favorite, YOU will love the perfume even more.

I know we wish we all had every single oil ever made, but alas, we don't. Or maybe one of your staples is out. I promise, it's okay to sub oils in for each other. You know that chart of notes back on page 19? Refer to that and choose a comparable oil and no one will ever know…and you might even love your newly chosen, *customized blend* even more!

CRYSTAL PAIRINGS

There are four main ways to put the crystals I recommend with each recipe to work with your oils!

1. Gemstone roller top

This is a roller top that is made out of an actual gemstone rather than glass, plastic, or stainless steel. Pop it onto your fav roller and ta-da! Crystal magic made easy.

2. Crystals inside your bottles

We make crystals tiny enough to fit inside of your bottles. They mix directly with the oils and are extra pretty in clear bottles. Add them into rollers, sprays, dropper blends for your diffuser, or anywhere else that needs a little crystal sprinkle.

3. Jewelry

Wear your favorite crystals and your favorite oils together. Diffusing jewelry is even better! There are lots of options, but my fav is faux suede. I've learned it holds the scent the longest.

4. Larger crystals

Crystals too big to fit in your bottles? These are perfect for decor, to hold while diffusing oils, or to take with you in a pocket or bag. Just having them in your home will induce smiles, which is a win.

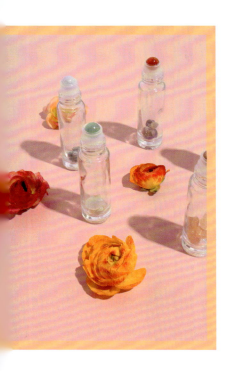

HOW TO MIX UP YOUR OILS

The numbers before each oil in the recipes represent how many drops of oil to put into that recipe.

My best tip for getting drops out is to be patient— hold the bottle of oil directly over the container you're adding them to, and wait for the drops to come. No need to shake or tap, they will come.

Oops, oils came out too fast and you got one too many in there? No stress! I promise, you can't mess this up.

RECIPES FOR DAYS

Emotions

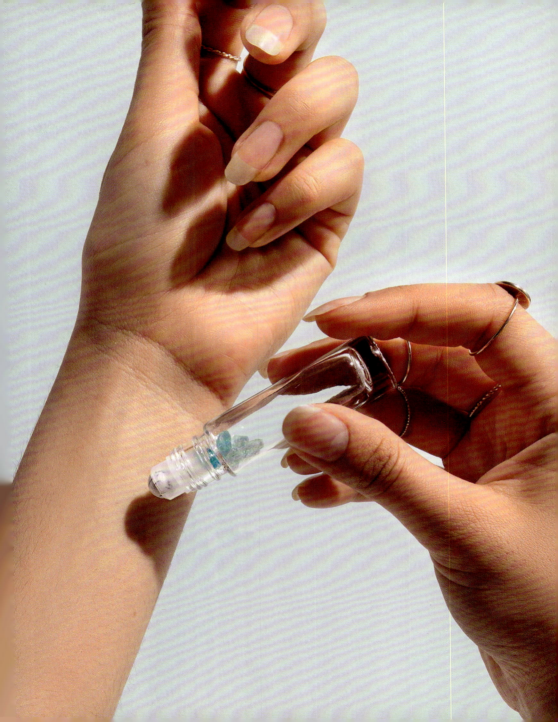

Emotions

peace roller blend

6 lavender + 5 bergamot +
3 fir + 2 sandalwood

Add drops to 10ml roller bottle, fill with carrier oil. Roll on neck and wrists to bring feelings of peace and grounding.

Pair with blue lace agate.

sunshine in my pocket diffuser blend

3 frankincense + 3 lavender + 3 orange

Add drops of oils to water in diffuser and breathe deeply.

Pair with sunstone.

happy happy happy roller blend

6 grapefruit + 4 fir + 2 lemon + 1 wintergreen

Add drops to 5ml roller bottle, fill with carrier oil. Roll on neck, wrists, and over heart for an uplifting feeling.

Pair with rhodonite.

zen baby roller blend

5 lavender + 3 orange + 2 vetiver

Add drops to 5ml roller bottle, fill with carrier oil. Roll on neck + wrists to help you unwind.

Pair with aquamarine.

i believe roller blend

3 frankincense + 4 orange + 2 cedarwood +
2 myrrh

Add drops to 5ml roller bottle, fill with carrier oil. Roll on heart and wrists to encourage meditation, insight, and prayer.

Pair with amethyst.

smile real big diffuser blend

4 citrus blend + 2 spearmint + 2 cedarwood +
2 jasmine

Add drops of oils to water in diffuser and breathe deeply.

Pair with citrine.

Whew. Feels are *real*. And they can get real big and real out of control real fast. Luckily, we've got oils and crystals! The oil blends and crystal pairings below utilize the science of aromatherapy, essential oils' proven therapeutic release, and traditional healing techniques to help you find your center again.

ROLL. DIFFUSE. FIND YOUR JOY AGAIN.

pixie dust roller blend

7 frankincense + 7 tangerine + 2 lemongrass + 3 lavender

Add drops to 10ml roller bottle, fill with carrier oil. Roll on neck and wrists to make you feel like you can fly! It's uplifting and energizing, a double whammy!

Pair with carnelian.

trust the process diffuser blend

5 fir + 3 bergamot + 3 frankincense + 1 ylang ylang

Add drops of oils to water in diffuser and breathe deeply.

Pair with clear quartz.

i wish (for no more laundry) roller blend

7 frankincense + 7 ylang ylang + 5 sandalwood + 5 patchouli

Add drops to 10ml roller bottle, fill with carrier oil. Roll on neck and wrists to give you hope.

Pair with garnet.

i am my favorite person perfume spray

18 sandalwood + 15 ylang ylang + 6 bergamot + 4 vetiver

Add drops to 1 oz spray bottle, then fill with vodka (witch hazel or water work too!). Shake well before each spray. Spritz yourself as you would with any perfume.

Pair with rose quartz.

hear me roar roller blend

10 grapefruit + 5 orange + 5 bergamot + 5 pine

Add drops to 10ml roller bottle, fill with carrier oil. Roll on neck and wrists when you need a confidence boost.

Pair with sunstone or tiger's eye.

chase the rainbow perfume spray

12 orange + 12 tangerine + 9 ylang ylang + 9 jasmine + 9 sandalwood

Add drops to 1 oz spray bottle, then fill with vodka (witch hazel or water work too!). Shake well and spritz yourself as you would with any perfume to bring out your inner child.

Pair with pink opal.

Spa vibes

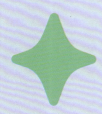

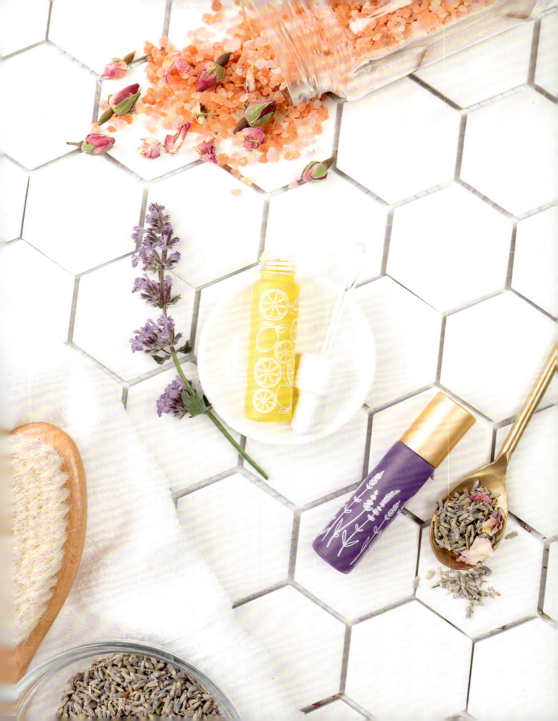

Spa vibes

softer than a baby's bottom body scrub

½ cup room temperature coconut oil + ¼ cup sugar + 5 drops orange + 5 drops lavender

Stir all ingredients together and store in an airtight container for 1 week.

Use as scrub wherever needed on your body.

mojito lip scrub

1 tbsp coconut oil (solid) + 1 tbsp honey + 2 tbsp brown sugar + 2 drops spearmint + 2 drops lime + 1 tsp vanilla extract

Mix honey, vanilla, essential oils, and coconut oil together until smooth. Add in brown sugar until combined. Rub on lips, then wipe off with warm washcloth. Store in fridge for up to two weeks.

better than botox facial spray

1/4 cup rose water + 4 drops lavender + 2 drops blue tansy

Add all ingredients to 2oz spray bottle. Shake well and spray on clean face.

i wish this bedroom was a spa linen spray

7 lavender + 5 eucalyptus + 3 cedarwood + 2 rosemary

Add drops to 2oz spray bottle, then fill with witch hazel, vodka, or water. Shake before each spray and spritz on any soft surface that needs refreshing.

rainbow diffuser blend

120 lemongrass + 90 spearmint + 60 bergamot

Add oils to a 15ml dropper bottle. Shake to combine. Add 5 drops into your diffuser, close your eyes, and pretend you're at the spa....

Pair with rainbow fluorite.

normal skin serum

10 frankincense + 6 geranium + 4 blue tansy

Add oils to 1oz dropper bottle and fill with jojoba oil. Use morning and/or night on a clean face. For extra moisture, top with your favorite moisturizer.

Pair with a jade facial roller for a delightful face massage.

Essential oils take me to another world. A whiff of the sugar scrub below, and I'm wrapped in a fluffy white robe, ready for my massage. The facial and linen sprays send me to sunlit fields in Tuscany, where there's no sound but the breeze running through the lavender. And you know what's absent in all of those magical essential oil worlds? Laundry.

dry skin serum

10 frankincense + 6 myrrh + 4 chamomile

Add oils to 1oz dropper bottle and fill with rosehip seed oil. Use morning and/or night on a clean face. For extra moisture, top with your favorite moisturizer.

Pair with a lapis lazuli facial roller for a delightful face massage.

oily or acne-prone skin serum

10 geranium + 6 patchouli + 4 lavender

Add oils to 1oz dropper bottle and fill with jojoba oil. Use morning and/or night on a clean face. I know it's weird I'm telling you to put oil on your oily skin, but trust me ;)

Pair with a rose quartz facial roller for a delightful face massage.

all the sleep you need glow serum

10 blue tansy + 7 frankincense + 5 copaiba

Add to roller bottle and fill with apricot kernel oil. Roll on face (avoiding eyes) every night for skin that looks like you got a full night's sleep (even if you didn't).

Pair with dalmatian stone.

the great outdoors is my spa diffuser blend

40 bergamot + 30 fir + 30 lavender + 30 eucalyptus

Add oils to 15ml dropper bottle and put 3-5 drops into your diffuser for a fresh, clean scent.

Pair with blue lace agate.

problems? what problems? bath salts blend

10 cardamom + 10 lavender + 10 tea tree

Add oils to 3 cups Epsom salt, 1 cup pink Himalayan salt, 1/2 cup baking soda, and up to 1 cup dried flowers (optional). Combine well and mix in hot water for a soothing bath.

Pair with pink opal.

nama stay zen diffuser blend

4 lavender + 3 frankincense + 2 sandalwood

Add water up to diffuser's fill line, and add oils.

Pair with clear quartz.

Love my body

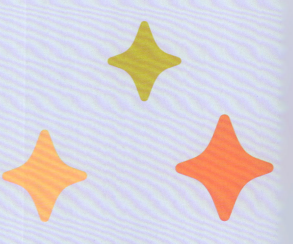

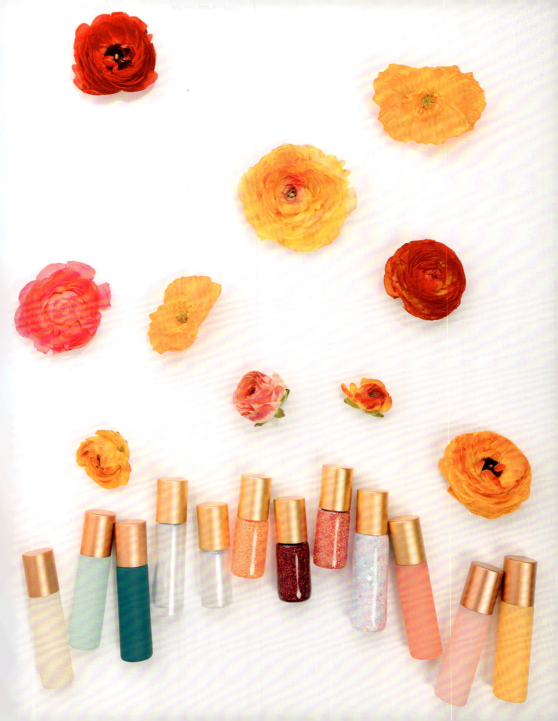

Love my body

i can do math in my head roller blend

5 peppermint + 5 rosemary + 3 lemon

Add drops to 5ml roller bottle, fill with carrier oil. Roll on neck or behind ears when you need help focusing.

Pair with rainbow fluorite.

moms don't get sick roller blend

8 frankincense + 6 lemon + 3 oregano

Add drops to 10ml roller bottle, fill with carrier oil. Roll on bottom of feet every day to support your immune system.

Pair with bloodstone.

breathing is nice roller blend

7 eucalyptus + 5 bay leaf (lauris nobilis) + 5 peppermint + 3 copaiba + 3 myrtle

Add drops to 10ml roller bottle, fill with carrier oil. Roll on neck and chest to help open airways.

Pair with green aventurine.

pepto but better roller blend

10 digestive blend + 5 peppermint + 3 ginger

Add drops to 10ml roller bottle, fill with carrier oil. Roll on tummy when it's feeling upset.

Pair with tiger's eye.

i work out roller blend

10 wintergreen + 5 helichrysum + 5 clove + 5 peppermint

Add drops to 10ml roller bottle, fill with carrier oil. Roll onto sore muscles.

Pair with hematite.

i dream of naps diffuser blend

30 cedarwood + 30 lavender + 15 chamomile + 13 vetiver

Add oils to a 15ml dropper bottle. Shake to combine. Add 5 drops into your diffuser before bed.

Pair with amethyst.

Oils and crystals are little earth geniuses when it comes to helping us connect to our bodies and live our brilliant, glorious lives. When has focusing ever been so delicious? Or sleep ever so dreamy? Or mornings ever so exciting and full of potential? And I can guarantee immunity-strengthening has *never* been this fun...

she fierce diffuser blend

30 citrus blend + 20 bergamot + 10 cinnamon + 5 peppermint

Add oils to 15ml dropper bottle. Shake to combine. Add drop 5-8 drops into diffuser in the morning to wake up and get ready for the day.

Pair with carnelian.

get my sleep on spray

20 lavender + 20 cedarwood + 10 frankincense

Add drops to a 2 oz spray bottle, then fill with witch hazel, vodka, or water. Shake before each spray and spritz your bed before climbing in at night.

I sing my own love songs roller blend

6 sandalwood + 5 ylang ylang + 2 bergamot + 1 vetiver

Add drops to 10ml roller bottle, fill with carrier oil. Roll over heart when you need to show yourself some love.

Pair with rose quartz.

skin magic roller blend

10 lavender + 5 copaiba + 5 frankincense

Add drops to 10ml roller bottle, fill with carrier oil. Roll where your skin needs extra healing.

Pair with jade.

give me energy roller blend

8 peppermint + 8 citrus blend + 2 nutmeg

Add drops to 10ml roller bottle, fill with carrier oil. Roll on neck and breathe deep for an energy boost.

Pair with carnelian.

everybody is stressin' me out roller blend

10 wintergreen + 5 helichrysum + 5 clove + 5 peppermint

Add drops to 10ml roller bottle, fill with carrier oil. Roll on area of body that's holding tension, avoiding eyes.

Pair with hematite.

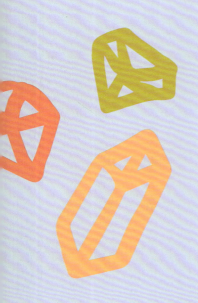

For him

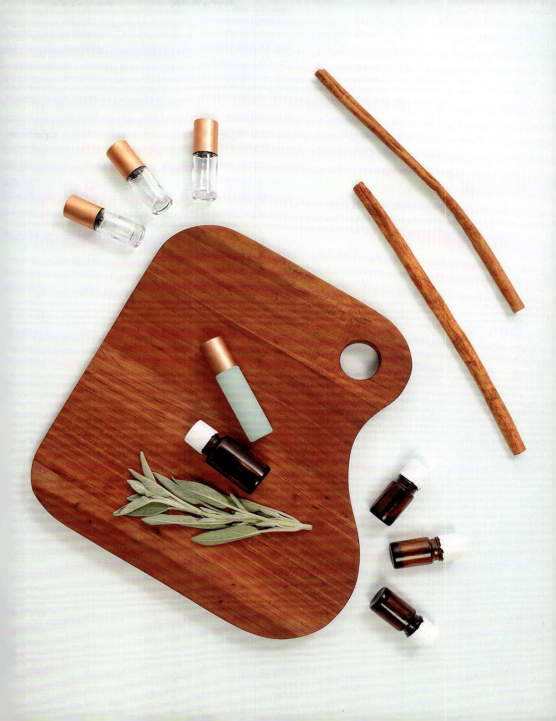

For him

best night's sleep of your life roller blend

10 lavender + 7 cedarwood + 3 orange

Add drops to 10ml roller bottle, fill with carrier oil. Roll on neck and wrists before bed to help you wind down and sleep.

Pair with hematite.

how you doin' cologne spray

12 cedarwood + 8 pine + 7 nutmeg + 6 clove + 4 lemon

Add drops to 15ml bottle and top with 100 proof (or higher) vodka or white rum. Spray on as cologne.

Pair with citrine.

manly man beard oil

4 cedarwood + 4 frankincense + 4 sandalwood

Add drops to 10ml dropper bottle and top with jojoba oil. Apply a few drops to your beard every day.

Pair with clear quartz.

working all day and night energy roller blend

6 orange + 5 frankincense + 2 patchouli + 2 nutmeg

Add drops to 10ml roller bottle, fill with carrier oil. Roll on neck as a motivating blend when you need to get things done.

Pair with carnelian.

who says men can't have spa days roller blend

5 lavender + 3 orange + 3 spruce + 2 vetiver

Add drops to 5ml roller bottle, fill with carrier oil. Roll on neck and wrists to help you unwind.

Pair with white howlite.

let's see those muscles roller blend

10 wintergreen + 5 helichrysum + 5 clove + 5 peppermint

Add drops to 10ml roller bottle, fill with carrier oil. Roll on sore muscles.

Pair with hematite.

We can't leave our men out from all this oily goodness. Sometimes he takes a little convincing before he's an oil convert—and sometimes he's all in before we are. Either way, he's going to love these calming, masculine scents for the impact they'll have on his sleep, focus, and muscle pain. And that cologne ain't half bad, either...

man flu roller blend

10 frankincense + 5 lemon + 4 clove + 2 oregano

Add drops to 10ml roller bottle, fill with carrier oil. Roll on the bottom of your feet everyday to boost your immune system.

Pair with clear quartz.

i'd rather be outside diffuser blend

5 fir + 4 spruce + 3 pine + 2 cedarwood

Add drops of oils to water in diffuser and enjoy the feeling of being deep in a pine forest —even when you're stuck at your computer.

Pair with aventurine.

big presentation vibes diffuser blend

7 grapefruit + 3 vetiver + 2 cedarwood + 2 sandalwood + 2 bergamot

Add drops of oils to water in diffuser and breathe deeply to calm nerves and increase focus.

Pair with citrine.

leave the work at the office diffuser blend

5 grapefruit + 4 eucalyptus + 3 patchouli

Add drops of oils to water in diffuser and breathe deeply to release the day's cares.

Pair with carnelian.

baths aren't just for girls bath salts blend

10 tea tree + 10 lavender + 10 grapefruit

Add oils to 3 cups Epsom salt and 1/2 cup baking soda. Combine well and mix in hot water for a soothing bath.

Pair with clear quartz.

my manly face needs soothing skin serum

8 lavender + 6 frankincense + 6 blue tansy

Add oils to 1oz dropper bottle and fill with jojoba oil. Use morning and/or night on a clean face. For extra moisture, top with your favorite moisturizer.

Pair with jade.

RECIPES FOR DAYS

For your littles

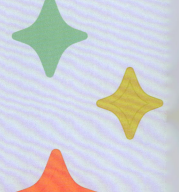

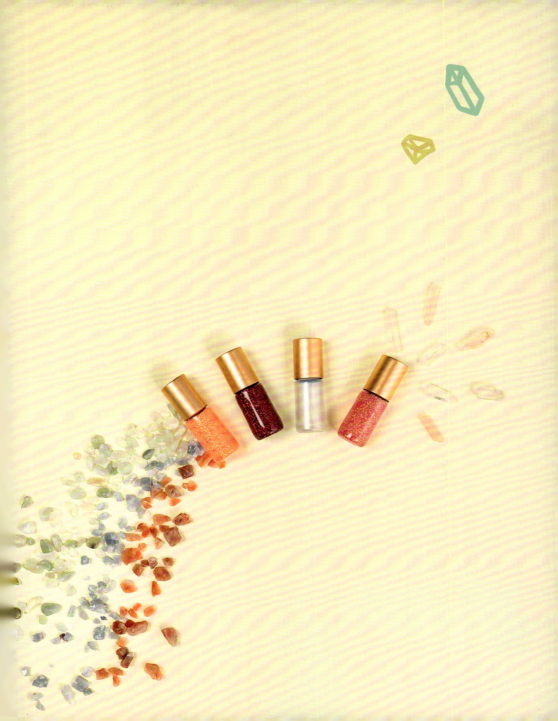

For your littles

please do your homework diffuser blend

40 peppermint + 25 rosemary + 30 lemon

Add oils to 15ml dropper bottle. Shake to combine. Add 3-6 drops to diffuser when your littles need to focus.

Pair with rainbow fluorite.

mommy needs you to go night night roller blend

3 lavender + 2 chamomile + 1 cedarwood

Add drops to 10ml roller bottle, fill with carrier oil. Use with littles ages 3+, dilute further for younger. Roll on neck before bed to help wind down.

Pair with amethyst.

we've lost that calm feeling roller blend

3 frankincense + 2 vetiver

Add drops to 10ml roller bottle, fill with carrier oil. Use with littles ages 3+, dilute further for younger. Roll on wrists for a calming feeling.

Pair with white howlite.

because i'm (trying to be) happy roller blend

3 frankincense + 2 grapefruit

Add drops to 10ml roller bottle, fill with carrier oil. Use with littles ages 3+, dilute further for younger. Roll on wrists for an uplifting scent.

Pair with rhodonite.

tummy probs roller blend

3 ginger + 2 spearmint

Add drops to 10ml roller bottle, fill with carrier oil. Use with littles ages 3+, dilute further for younger. Roll on tummy when it's feeling upset.

Pair with tiger's eye.

no sick here roller blend

3 frankincense + 2 oregano

Add drops to 10ml roller bottle, fill with carrier oil. Use with littles ages 3+, dilute further for younger. Roll on bottom of feet everyday to support immune system.

Pair with clear quartz.

These days, I spell relief O-I-L-S! It's seriously the best to have help for my kids that's non-toxic and doesn't have any weird or dangerous side effects. These blends are my ride or dies—keep them ready on the draw for everything from bug bites to upset tummies to big feels to homework torture to sleep troubles. You can thank me later. Now if only there was an oil to teach kids how to pick up after themselves...

some dadgum peace & quiet diffuser blend

4 peace blend + 2 lavender

Add drops of oils to water in diffuser when your home needs some chill.

Pair with amazonite.

no more monsters under the bed room spray

6 bergamot + 4 ylang ylang + 3 myrrh + 3 geranium + 2 sandalwood

Add oils to 1 oz spray bottle and fill with witch hazel or water. Shake well before each spray and let your little spray under the bed and in the closet to scare those monsters away!

Pair with tourmaline.

we're both learning here diffuser blend

30 lavender + 20 clary sage + 30 roman chamomile

Add oils to 15ml dropper bottle. Shake to combine. Add 3-6 drops to a diffuser for support when you bring a new baby home.

Pair with rose quartz.

better baby diaper rash cream

3 lavender + 3 chamomile

Add oils to 1/8 cup organic virgin coconut oil and 1/8 cup organic raw grade A shea butter and mix well. Apply to baby's clean bottom after a diaper change to prevent or heal diaper rash.

teeth are the worst roller blend

2 Roman chamomile + 2 lavender + 2 copaiba

Add drops to 15ml roller bottle, fill with carrier oil. Roll gently on jawline when baby is teething.

Pair with topaz.

the magic wand roller blend

3 lavender + 2 tea tree

Add drops to 15ml roller bottle, fill with carrier oil. Roll gently on bug bites or owies for immediate relief.

Pair with amethyst.

Seasons

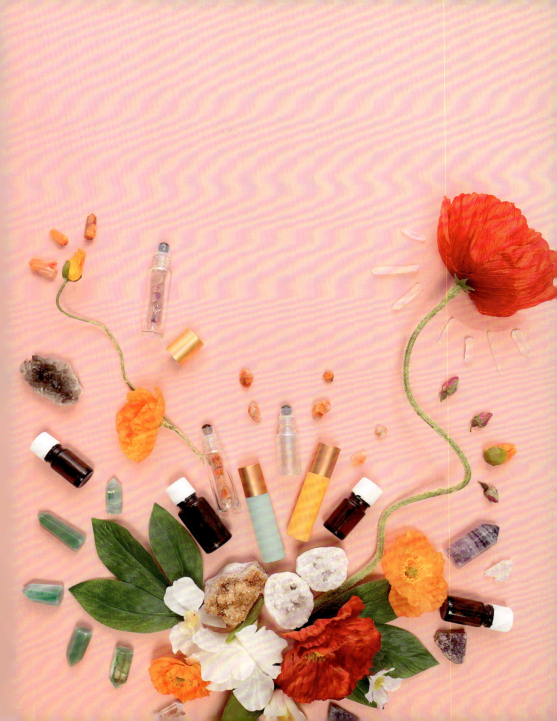

RECIPES FOR DAYS

Seasons: Spring

There's some serious wisdom in the earth's seasons, and I find myself reaching for my oils and crystals at the turn of each to help me lean into whatever's happening: new life in the spring, fun and adventure in the summer, connection and coziness in the fall, and rest and stillness in the winter.

Try the blends and prepare to open up your heart and home to all that lovely goodness each season serves up.

bye pollen roller blend

4 lavender + 4 peppermint + 4 lemon

Add drops to 5ml roller bottle, fill with carrier oil. Roll on neck and near sinuses (avoiding eyes) during seasonal changes.

Pair with aventurine.

extra flowers please perfume spray

15 lavender + 10 ylang ylang + 10 lime + 5 geranium

Add drops to 1 oz spray bottle, then fill with vodka (witch hazel or water work too!). Shake well before each spray. Spritz yourself to be reminded of fresh cut blooms.

Pair with amethyst.

perky diffuser blend

2 orange + 3 frankincense + 2 peppermint

Add water up to diffuser's fill line, and add oils.

Pair with rhodonite.

how does your garden grow spray

50 peppermint

Add drops to 8oz spray bottle the fill with water. Shake well and spray on garden leaves to get rid of pesky creatures.

Pair with your favorite garden rock to make you smile while gardening.

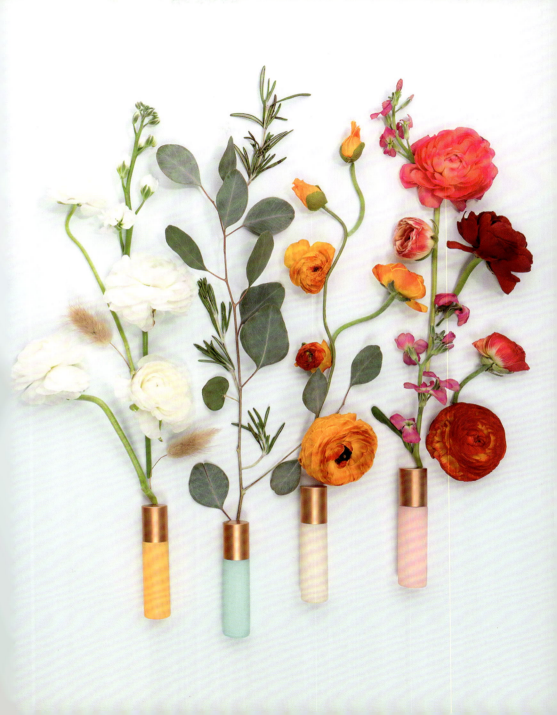

Seasons: Summer

calm down, sun spray

12 lavender + 12 chamomile

Add drops to 2oz spray bottle. Fill with witch hazel and shake before each spray. Spritz on skin after spending too much time in the sun.

Pair with amethyst.

ahhhhh cooling mist

15 peppermint + 10 lavender

Fill 2oz bottle with water and oils; spray on skin when you need to cool down.

Pair with chrysocolla.

bug off spray

15 lemongrass + 15 eucalyptus + 20 citronella

Add drops to 4oz spray bottle. Fill with witch hazel and shake before each spray; spray on skin before venturing outside.

Pair with smoky quartz

tgi summer diffuser blend

3 ylang ylang + 3 grapefruit + 3 sandalwood + 1 lime

Add water up to diffuser's fill line, and add oils.

Pair with amethyst.

vacation in a bottle roller blend

5 orange + 4 vanilla + 4 lime + 2 cedarwood

Add drops to 10ml roller bottle, fill with carrier oil. Roll on neck and wrists and pretend you are on a beach somewhere.

Pair with citrine.

s'mores diffuser blend

5 vetiver + 2 cedarwood + 2 copaiba + 2 vanilla + 2 orange

Add water up to diffuser's fill line, and add oils.

Pair with tourmaline.

Seasons: Fall

omg it's fall diffuser blend

40 cinnamon + 30 cardamom + 30 orange + 30 clove

Add oils to 15ml dropper bottle. Shake to combine. Add 5 drops to diffuser for that flannels and scarves feeling.

Pair with smoky quartz.

spicy spray

7 spruce + 5 cinnamon + 5 clove + 3 nutmeg + 3 cardamom

Add drops to 2oz spray bottle and top with witch hazel, vodka, or water. Shake before each spray and spritz anywhere for a spicy scent boost.

Pair with hematite.

i love this home diffuser blend

2 orange + 2 clove + 1 spruce + 1 cinnamon

Add water up to diffuser's fill line, and add oils for a scent that will remind you of crisp leaves and a cozy home.

Pair with citrine.

zen & cozy roller blend

6 lavender + 5 bergamot + 3 fir + 2 sandalwood

Add drops to 10ml roller bottle, fill with carrier oil. Roll on neck and wrists and breathe deeply.

Pair with smoky quartz.

make me smell like pumpkin spice roller blend

3 clove + 3 cinnamon + 2 nutmeg + 2 orange + 1 ginger

Add drops to 10ml roller bottle, fill with carrier oil. Roll on neck and wrists while you drink your PSL.

Pair with tiger's eye.

be well, my friend diffuser blend

4 frankincense + 3 lemon + 2 eucalyptus

Add water up to diffuser's fill line, and add oils for a scent that will clear the air.

Pair with amethyst.

Seasons: Winter

treat every day like christmas roller blend

6 orange + 4 sandalwood + 3 clove +
2 cinnamon + 1 patchouli

Add drops to 10ml roller bottle, fill with
carrier oil. Roll on neck and wrists for a
warming and spicy scent.

Pair with smoky quartz.

new year, i'm perfect perfume spray

4 orange + 4 tangerine + 3 ylang ylang +
3 jasmine + 3 sandalwood

Add drops to 10ml spray bottle, fill with
vodka, water or witch hazel. Spray on for a
sultry and playful scent.

Pair with ruby.

jingle all the way roller blend

10 grapefruit + 5 orange + 5 bergamot +
5 pine

Add drops to 10ml roller bottle, fill with carrier
oil. Roll on neck and wrists for a happy scent.

Pair with garnet.

lights diffuser blend

35 vanilla extract or oil + 20 orange +
16 clove + 10 cinnamon

Add oils to 15ml dropper bottle. Shake
to combine. Add 3-5 drops to diffuser for
feelings of warmth + coziness.

Pair with rose quartz.

ya'll, it's cold out there diffuser blend

2 fir + 2 peppermint + 1 wintergreen

Add water up to diffuser's fill line, and add in oils.

Pair with smoky quartz.

i'm not a baker (but i play one on tv) diffuser blend

4 orange + 3 clove + 2 nutmeg + 2 ginger

Add water up to diffuser's fill line, add oils,
and make your house smell like you've been
baking all day.

Pair with tiger's eye.

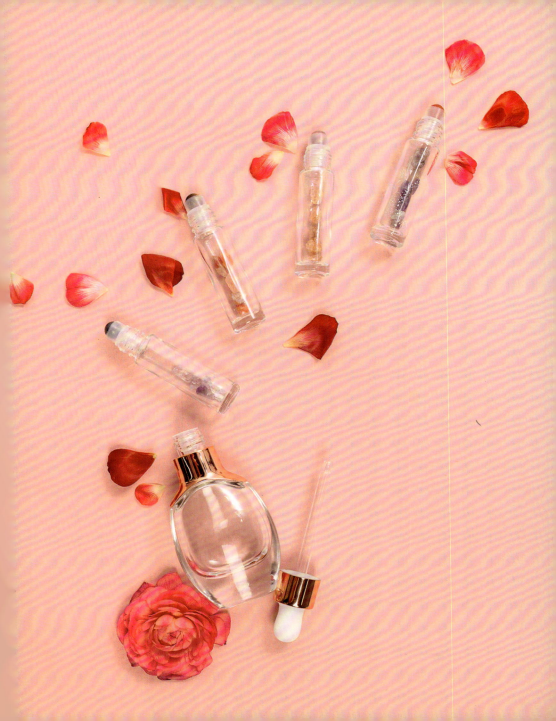

RECIPES FOR DAYS

Home

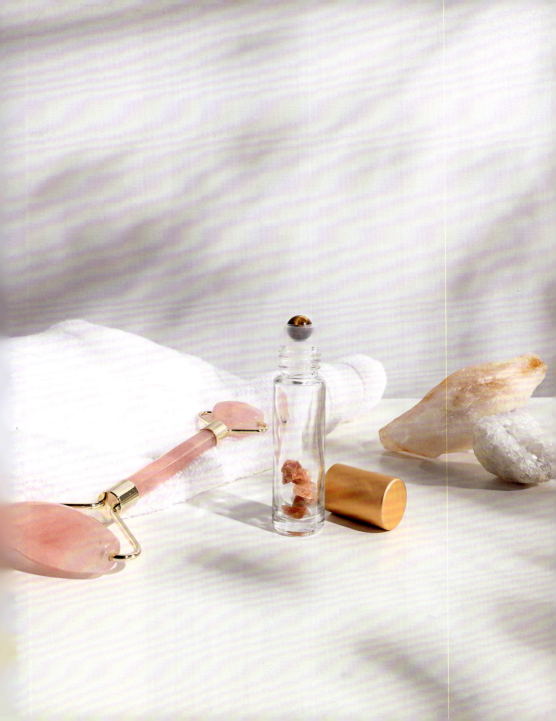

Home

no more finger (or paw) prints glass cleaner

1/4 c. white vinegar + 1 tbsp cornstarch + 1 3/4 cups warm water + 20 drops lemon

Mix all ingredients in a 16oz spray bottle, shake well. Spray on windows, mirrors, or anything else that needs some sparkle and wipe dry!

let's pretend the carpet guys came carpet refresher

1 cup of baking soda + 10 drops lemon

Mix baking soda and oils together, sprinkle all over your carpet, let sit for 20 minutes, then vacuum it up!

wash your hands foaming hand soap

3/4 cup castile soap + 1 tbsp jojoba, vitamin e, or olive oil (helps nourish skin) + 5 drops orange

Grab yourself a foaming soap dispenser (feel free to reuse here!) and add ingredients. Fill the container with water gently so it doesn't create tons of bubbles. Pair with your fave crystal by your sink to stare at while you wash up.

too many zoom meetings diffuser blend

5 peppermint + 3 rosemary + 3 lemon

Add water up to diffuser's fill line, and add in oils, breathe deeply and try to focus.

Pair with rainbow fluorite.

i just "cleaned" my house diffuser blend

40 lemongrass + 30 spearmint + 20 lemon

Add oils to 15ml dropper bottle and put 3-5 drops into your difuser of this blend for a fresh scent.

Pair with selenite.

i dream in rainbows linen spray

21 bergamot + 15 spruce + 9 lemon + 6 rosemary

Fill a 2oz bottle with witch hazel or vodka and shake before each spray. Spray on any soft surface that needs refreshing.

Ah, home. That magical place where everybody gets along, I'm always able to focus, and unicorns play happily in the corner. Wait—what? Not my home! Messes + squabbles and big feelings + mama trying to get some work done is more like it! That's why I need my oils—and why I created these fantastic home recipe blends. You'll love them. Unless you do have unicorns, in which case, hit me up.

coming up lemons counter top spray

10 cinnamon + 10 tea tree + 10 lemon

Combine oil, 2oz white vinegar, and 14oz distilled water to 16oz glass spray bottle. Shake to combine and use as counter top spray or all purpose cleaner.

Pair with citrine.

let's rinse that first produce wash

2 drops lemon essential oil + 5-6 drops castile soap

Fill clean sink with water, and add soap and oil. Add produce, and let sit for ten minutes. Rinse produce, and dry; your fruits & veggies should last longer now!

bye, mystery smell diffuser blend

25 lemon + 20 rosemary +20 tea tree + 15 lavender + 10 lemongrass + 10 myrtle

Add oils to 15ml dropper bottle and put 3-5 drops into your diffuser to knock out bad odors. You can also add 40 drops of this blend to a 2oz spray bottle and top with witch hazel to create a room spray.

Pair with selenite.

that candle (you know the one) diffuser blend

50 grapefruit + 50 orange + 40 lime + 30 geranium + 30 blue spruce

Add oils to 15ml dropper bottle and put 3-5 drops into your diffuser when you want your home to smell like your favorite store.

Pair with smoky quartz.

we so bougie diffuser blend

5 northern lights black spruce + 5 bergamot + 5 patchouli

Add oils to diffuser, top with water, and diffuse for a mysteriously unexpected combination.

Pair with carnelian.

tastes like cotton candy diffuser blend

20 ylang ylang + 30 grapefruit + 10 vanilla

Add oils to 15ml dropper bottle and put 3-5 drops into your diffuser for an almost edible experience.

Pair with amazonite.

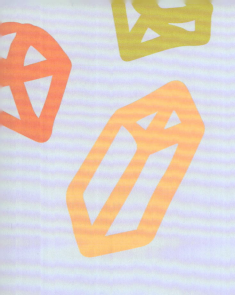

My happy place

ALL THE THINGS I CAN'T FORGET TO TELL YOU

No way around it: the more we use essential oils, the more they'll help us. Here are my final two cents on squeezing all that juicy goodness from your lemons—er—oils:

DO THIS RIGHT THIS SECOND

Stop and do not pass go until you've whipped up two or three of your favorite recipes from this book. Don't overthink it. Sub in an oil you have for one you don't have if you need to. At the very least, choose two recipes you want to make and order the supplies. Go, I'm waiting.

Smiling is a great thing

If an oil's aroma makes you smile whenever you walk by your diffuser, or a crystal makes you grin when you see it on your shelf—well, isn't that a win? Sometimes I waaaay over complicate things and I always remind myself: if we're smiling, we're winning.

I feel pretty

Am I the only one who thinks it works better when it's in a prettier package? I'm not the type to judge a book by its cover, but I am the type to use my oils more when they're in pretty bottles. I mean that's literally why I started Whimsy + Wellness. So go now, and buy some pretty bottles. I promise you're worth it.

TELL ME ABOUT IT, GIRL!

I'm just a girl, in her office, with three kids, wondering how I'm going to get it all done. You know what I live for? YOU!

Your emails, Instagram tags, and messages letting me know what a difference Whimsy + Wellness is making in your life light up my heart like none other! Post about this book or your favorite recipes and don't forget to tag me. We are 100% on this whimsical wellness adventure together!

Cheers to more whimsy,

Haylee

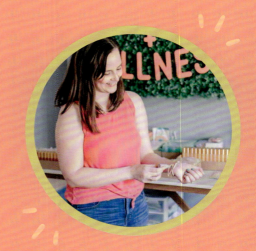

ACKNOWLEDGEMENTS

roll. smile. repeat.

For my husband, Russ. You cheered me on from day one and never doubted that I could build this business. When I asked if we could spend money on vinyl, then roller bottles, then a printer. . . the list goes on and your answer was always YES.
Whimsy + Wellness would not be what it is without you.

I love you more than you know.

And I guess I should also mention our kids here, huh? :)

Mason, Posey, and Golden.
We work hard for you. I hope you know that you can achieve anything you put your mind to. You see it every day watching your dad and I work. We love you more than you know.

© 2020 Haylee Crowley

notes

notes

notes

notes

notes

notes

notes

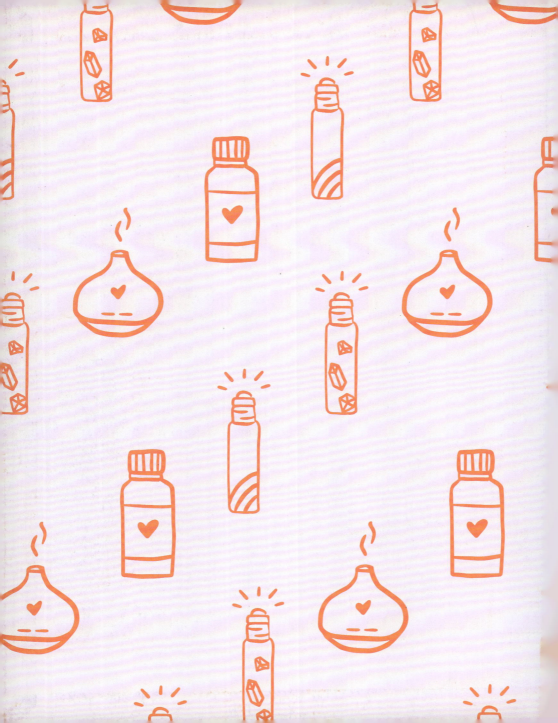